EARLY CAREER

IN

PUBLIC HEALTH

Adanze Nge Cynthia

1

Contact author:

Email: ngecynthia22@gmail.com

Facebook: Cynthia Nge

Linkedin: Adanze Nge Cynthia

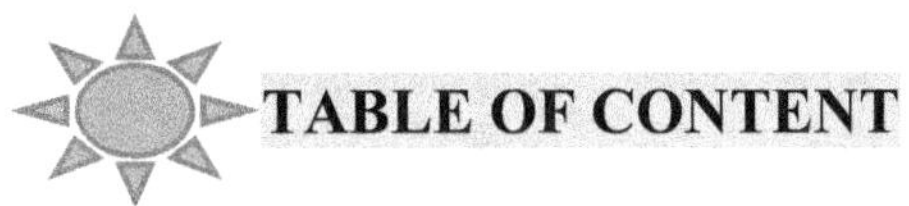 **TABLE OF CONTENT**

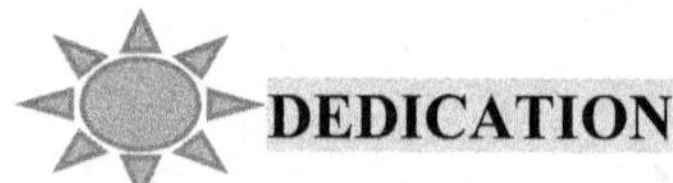 **DEDICATION**

This book is dedicated to all those considering pursuing a career in Public Health for the first time and also for early-career public health experts.

It is also dedicated to all those who are about to venture into any professional field and have doubts

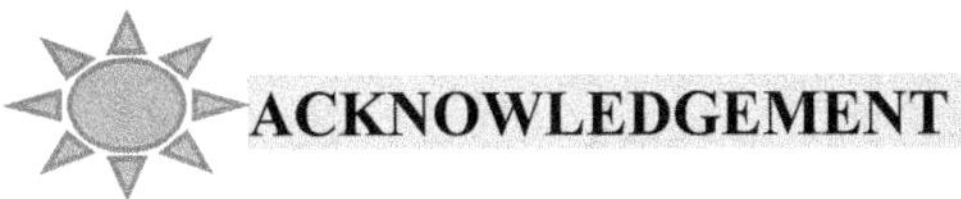

ACKNOWLEDGEMENT

I want to thank my family, especially my parents; Madam Abunaw Pauline Enow and Dr. Raymond Chinedum Nge for investing their time, energy, and resources in educating and supporting me. I am grateful for the sacrifices you continue to play in my career journey.

A big thank you to Chiara Fenangi, for always lending a helping hand despite her own busy schedule.

To the entire staff of the University of Buea, both the Faculty of Science, Department of Microbiology and Parasitology, and Faculty of Health Sciences, Department of Public Health and Hygiene, I appreciate the pedagogic efforts made in shaping the person I am today. To the University of Buea, Faculty of Health Sciences, MPH graduating class of 2018, thank you for inspiring me to write this book based on our experiences.

 To the proofreading team; Dr. Frankline S. Wirsey, and Dickson Ndzi, thank you for the sacrifice of time and the useful remarks and edits. Thank you to all of my mentees. You are one of the most important motivators for this book. To my friends and well-wishers, who have in one way or another other shared their support either financially, morally, or physically, I say thank you.

Finally, last but in no way least, my sincere gratitude to God Almighty, the giver of all knowledge and wisdom, for the inspiration to write this book.

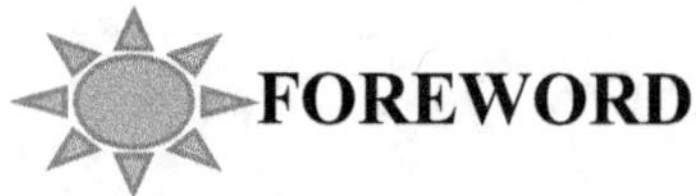# FOREWORD

Without a doubt, public health ia a rapidly growing field with many people gaining interest in it. Heading the Department of Public Health and Hygiene, University of Buea, for many years, I have seen many of my students begin as fresh naive public health scholars and graduate as young career public health experts.The book EARLY CAREER IN PUBLIC HEALTH by Cynthia Adanze Nge is not only timely but very informative to those thinking of venturing into the field of public health.

With the flip of every page in this book, I found myself unconsciously nodding in total agreement with the ideas presented. Summarizing from her own personal narrative of how she found herself in the public health field, the realities on the ground, the challenges, and advice on how to overcome the challenges. This book is indeed a masterpiece for those considering public health as a career and also for early starters in the public health sector.

Writing is difficult even for those who do it frequently, so Adanze's ability to write this eloquently yet in very simple, realistic, and easily understandable terms is highly commendable. If you have the desire to pursue a career in public health or are an early career public health practitioner or wish to know what is all about public health, then this book is for you. I fully recommend this book to you.

Dr. Tendongfor Nicholas
Medical Microbiologist/Public Health Biostatistician
Head of Department of Public Health and Hygiene,
Faculty of Health Sciences,
The University of Buea

CHAPTER 1

HOW I FOUND MYSELF IN THE FIELD OF PUBLIC HEALTH

One question comes up time and time again, whether it is from people I mentor, those who seek me out for help with continuing their education, or friends and acquaintances. The following is the question:

Why did you choose to do public health?

This specific question usually makes me grin before I respond, especially when I notice the expectant expression on the faces of people who are asking, evidently waiting for the perfect answer (smiles). I'll stutter at first, trying to think of a more appealing way to say the "not so expected response" so as not to disappoint them. But today, with the experiences and positive feedback I have gotten, I tell those who ask the answer in a short story. Permit me to tell you a little bit about how I came to work in this particular field. Freshly graduated with a Bachelor of Science in Microbiology with a minor in Medical Laboratory Sciences, there was this vast sea of confusion.

I was unsure if I should work or pursue a Master's degree, and if so, what specialty or area, as some people call it? Yes, I liked Microbiology, but with the few laboratories I had worked in, I didn't have a strong conviction to pursue a Master's degree in that field. Furthermore, to be quite honest, when I looked at the salary package of a Microbiologist or Laboratory technician at the time, it was uninspiring.

In Cameroon after graduation from undergraduate studies, you are faced with a lack of a job or a very competitive job market, and the instant you secure one, so many things are required of you, either directly or indirectly (Sako, 2011). I frequently admire my older sister, who is an excellent laboratory technician, but I felt deep down that I wouldn't be as good as she is since I was not convinced it was where I wanted to be. Let's take a pause from my story to highlight a few points. I did not choose to specialize full-time in Microbiology not because it's a sub-standard field or because there are fewer opportunities there.

The truth is that many Microbiologists and Laboratory Technicians I know are financially secure and highly successful in their fields. My lack of interest prevented me from exploring further choices or piqued my interest in figuring out how to make a living in that sector. Not everyone can be a Microbiologist or a Laboratory Technician, and not everyone can be a Public Health Expert.

Back to my story.

So, after graduation, I went home still grossly confused. I was about to leave on a vacation when I learned that the university where I just graduated had launched a Master's program in both Epidemiology and Public Health and was receiving applications.

My very close friend and I talked about the launch of these two programs (Epidemiology and Public Health) but had not settled on which one to do. The debate about whether it should be Epidemiology or Public Health went back and forth among us, with none of us knowing why we should select one over the other (laughs).

It was not until she told me;

"Ada, you know what? I guess I'll go for public health."

I remained silent for a while, knowing that if I asked why we would go back and forth again. When I informed my mother, she questioned whether I was sure that was the right choice for me. I nodded, though I still did not understand why I made that choice, or better still, I couldn't tell her exactly how my choice was made.

Mind you, public health was still not a profession that many people in my country were familiar with, let alone aspired to explore. Like many others, I had scarcely heard someone announce themselves as "I am a public health expert, public health specialist, or public health personnel," but I knew Epidemiologists existed.

So, I enrolled in the Master of Public Health program, often known as MPH, and submitted all of the required documentation alongside my friend and I jetted off on holidays.

While on vacation, we were encouraged to keep
an eye out for probable selection announcements on the university's website.

So, on that particular day, I received a whatsapp message from my friend containing a screenshot of the list of those selected for the MPH program. We had both been chosen, and I was overjoyed. It's funny since I still did not know why I was getting into public health at this time.

The story gets better because this is not the end (smiles). I cut short my holidays and returned home to complete all university enrolment requirements. The next lines you will be reading in this story of mine are the perfect answers to the question ''why did you choose public health or why are you so passionate about public health?''.

We had numerous professors attend our first class and give the customary first-class introductions. There was this speaker who, unbeknownst to him, is the reason I am firmly anchored in public health. He was an old and knowledgeable professor of the subject.

He requested us to identify ourselves as follows: "your name, your undergraduate degree, and why you picked public health."

I enjoyed sitting in the back. So, while some of my classmates struggled to answer the question, others who knew everything astonished the class with their responses, and then it was my turn.

I was already sweating and feeling palpitations (laughs) since I knew I could not explain exactly why I selected public health to him. I stuttered as I explained why I picked public health, and I recall him telling me to pause (clearly perplexed and knowing I did not know why I was in that class) and asking me;
'What is the current life expectancy of Cameroonians?' What is the birth and death rate in Cameroon, and what are the top five diseases?'
At this exact point in time, my frustration was very evident.

Not only did I not have a good justification for choosing public health, but I was also naive about the most fundamental national data. Then, in a firm yet fatherly tone, he addressed the class:

"When you return home today, consider why you are in the area of public health; this will influence how far and how successful you will go in this profession."

I still remember when my friend and I were walking back home that day, as we normally did, I was quite quiet and in a deep-thinking mood, unlike previous days when I would always laugh loudly while conversing. We parted ways, and I returned home with mixed thoughts two questions kept coming to my mind:

Was it deliberate? Was my ignorance so visible from afar or why did that professor lecturer single me out to ask the most challenging of questions?

Those questions felt like an attack on me back then. I recall frowning and asking myself, "Am I a magician to know all those figures?" Today, knowing these facts not only seems normal to me but keeps me on my toes as well as the tendencies that underlie these facts.

Why did I choose public health?

The second question is why I am writing this book now and what my story and ongoing public health journey are all about.

I went to Google without even thinking about it or defending my lack of knowledge at the moment. I remember doing a number of searches, some of which I will share with you the reader in the hopes of eradicating some of the confusion you may be experiencing at the moment.

I researched the following topics;

- Who is a public health specialist?
- What are the sub-branches or specializations under public health?
- How do they call someone who did public health (like a professional title)

- What are the career prospects in Cameroon for someone working in public health? (Because I am a Cameroonian, you may substitute with your nationality.)
- What are the career prospects for someone working in public health in other parts of the world? (Substitute the world with the countries you wish to work in)
- Will public health remain a thriving career in the next ten to twenty years?
- What types of organizations or businesses do public health professionals work for?
- How much does a public health specialist make on average in Cameroon and other countries?

Those were a handful of the questions I posed to myself. The more I looked, the clearer I became of the field in which I was previously a novice. When I was done, I recalled a surge of confidence and contentment washing over me. It was as if I had discovered a treasure lying in the depths of the ocean. Yes, I did not and still do not fully understand public health in its entirety because, like any other field, things always change, but I was aware of the reasons for my desire to work in this field. When I learned the explanations, they matched not just my personal and humanitarian goals but also my professional aspirations.

That is the story of how I found myself in the field of public health.

Despite the fact that I have not spent decades in this sector, I am certain that this is where I am intended to be.

Each time I finish relating the tale of how I ended up in the field of public health, the most common responses I hear are;

" We have no doubt that you are genuinely enthusiastic about what you do"

"You make public health appear so simple (I always smile at this particular comment because the reality is, nothing is easy but with the right fortitude, you will find ease out of every difficulty)"

"I'd want to have you as a mentor since I'd like to work in public health but don't believe I'm qualified."

One of the remarks I occasionally hear is, "Ada, you are the one who inspired me to venture into the field of public health." As much as I am pleased to have inspired you to pursue a career in public health, I hope you find the proper reasons to stay motivated in the area.

Without your personal findings and drive to pursue a career in public health, my narrative may not equip you with the fortitude and grit to face the severe winds.

Self-reflection questions

A. *For individuals considering a career in public health, ask yourself:*

i. Why exactly do I want to pursue public health?

Ii. Have I done enough personal research and do I have enough information on public health?

B. *For those who are currently in the field, consider the following questions:*

What additional skills or courses do I need to pursue in order to enhance my public health career?

How well informed am I about everyday changes in my domain?

With everyone getting into public health, how can I stay relevant?

These are questions for self-reflection. I ask myself these questions frequently, and if I see a knowledge debt or a familiarity crisis, I strive to overcome it. These issues apply not only to the field of public health but to any other specialty in which you may find yourself.

CHAPTER 2

IDENTITY CONFLICT IN THE PUBLIC HEALTH FIELD

'Belonging is a widely undervalued condition required for human performance' Owen Eastwood

Identity crises, like any other aspect of life, are very visible and can be problematic if not handled carefully (Elmer, 2019). I'm sure you're wondering what kind of identity crises could exist in the field of public health.

Not to worry, this chapter will highlight some of the identity crises that may arise in this field and how to possibly resolve them.

We will examine this identity conflict from two perspectives: before entering the field and while you are in the field.

Perspective 1: Identity Conflict Before Entering the Field

Let's go over how I ended up in the field of public health again. Microbiology was my undergraduate major.

The "crowd opinions" were one barrier that made me unsure whether to pursue public health or not. I call them crowd opinions because they frequently contain little truth.

"You cannot do an MPH if you studied microbiology," said the majority of the audience.

Because they are the same thing, you must be a medical doctor to specialize in MPH (whenever I hear such now, I always laugh out because the reality is this; there is a big difference between public health and medicine which we will discuss in detail in this chapter).

Before you can pursue an MPH, you must have 5 years of work experience. The MPH program is only available to science majors.

There are many other crowd opinions, but we will concentrate on the ones mentioned above. Many people have missed out on opportunities due to a lack of information and the power of crowd opinion.

Although some crowd opinions may be correct, relying on such information to make important decisions such as a career path is strongly discouraged.

We live in a world where changes occur on a daily basis. Always seek information from reputable sources, and remember each university may have different requirements. What is required for a university in Cameroon may not be required for a university in Nigeria or another country?

If you completed an undergraduate course in Microbiology or another science-related course and are interested in pursuing a career in public health, GO FOR IT! Do your research and don't let the opinions of the crowd get the best of you. Most people who claim it's impossible to have either never attempted enrolment, but were deemed ineligible or simply heard from other people that it's not possible.

Do thorough research before giving up on your dream due to crowd opinion. Crowd opinions may be a contributing factor but do not let it be the sole determining reason.

Another crowd opinion that may cause you to doubt your readiness for a career in public health is a lack of experience. Yes, in the past, especially in my country, candidates willing to pursue a Master's degree in any field, not just public health, were expected to have worked for some number of years.But that is no longer the case. Most universities welcome students who want to pursue a career in a field of their choice without the burden of years of experience.

You will gain the necessary experience even while still in school. So, don't let a lack of experience make you question whether you're ready to pursue a career in MPH. If you can gain some work experience (volunteering included) before pursuing a career in public health, that is ideal, but if you cannot, don't let that deter you.

Then, there was the misconception that public health was only for science majors, which was incorrect.

As unlikely as it may seem to most of you, public health is most often seen as a social science (Dhakal, 2020). In more simple terms, most, if not all, disciplines can pursue a degree in public health when viewed holistically.

I frequently advise people who ask me if they can pursue a career in public health to first understand what public health is. If you've ever wondered, the definition states unequivocally that public health is both a science and an art. So, if you are reading this and are in the arts sector, you will find your identity in public health with the right guidance and motivation.

Perspective 2: Identity Conflict After Entering the Field

One would think that after finally surviving the storms and entering the field of public health, everything would fall into place (smiles). That may not be the case, especially since some people do not fully comprehend how the field of public health works.

I once found myself in a very awkward situation. I ran to a friend of mine who was out with two of her friends, a man and a woman in their late thirties. My friend introduced me as a public health specialist after the introductions were made. "Oh, so you're a medical doctor," the man said right away. I smiled and replied, "no, sir, I am not, I am a public health specialist." I could see the confusion on their faces right away. The man tried so hard to hide it, but the lady, unable to conceal her confusion any longer, asked me with great uncertainty, "if you are pursuing a Ph.D. in public health, it means you have previously studied medicine and public health your specialty?"

I smiled and said, *"No, ma'am, I am not a medical doctor, but a soon-to-be Doctor of Public Health."*

It was very clear that neither of them could comprehend how I could be doing public health without a medical background. I wanted to explain, but time was against me. I'm not sure if this experience is unique to me, but I've heard a few of my colleagues express their dissatisfaction with this identity conflict.

It is important to note that there is a significant distinction between a public health specialist and a medical doctor. In very simple terms, one of my professors during my MPH program would frequently say;

''Medicine is one-on-one people-centered whereas public health is community centered''

Although it is easy to assume that because public health contains the word "health," it is most likely for scientists, keep in mind that the word "public" is the game changer.

In my early career, I was often discouraged or intimidated when someone looked disappointed when I explained that I am not a medical doctor but a public health expert.

Nowadays, I am surprised and always tease such people about how they do not know about an important and relevant title like "public health specialist."So, whether you're just starting a career in public health or you've been in the field for a while, if you come across such situations, develop an anti-shock or anti-provocation mechanism, because many people still do not know the difference. Rather than becoming enraged, if you have the time, educate them on the distinction, emphasizing how unbalanced the world would be without public health specialists like ourselves (smiles).

Being undervalued or misunderstood can cause one to doubt themselves not only in the public health domain but in all aspects of life.

Although public health is on the rise with many people aware of its importance and its unique roles and responsibilities, many people do not fully comprehend the role of a public health expert. Another major identity crisis in this field is the question of what exactly is my professional title.

Even while it seems funny, it is actually rather challenging, especially when you are in a professional setting and need to introduce yourself.

We created a class whatsapp group to facilitate information flow when I was doing my MPH. Years after graduation, this group still serves other purposes, such as marriage and birth announcements, scholarship opportunities for those wishing to further their education, and, most importantly, job opportunities. During one of the discussions, a colleague of ours brought to the class's attention a problem he was having. He asked;

''Course mates I have a question it may seem funny but what exactly is our title? What do you write when applying for jobs, as a title when attending conferences or professional gatherings, or even when introducing yourself?"

The responses made us laugh because almost all of us could attest to the fact that we had either experienced or are still battling with what title best fits us.

Some claimed to be public health experts, while others claimed to be public health specialists.

Others claimed to be public health personnel, while only one claimed to have simply added the degree title, MPH, to the end of their names.

Whether or not our colleague had found the perfect title for himself, one thing was certain: we were all facing the same problem. Someone confided in me that she was afraid to refer to herself as a public health expert because she felt she was too young and had not gained enough experience. She solemnly stated that such a prestigious title was reserved for those who had been in the field for at least 20 years. This is someone I know who is more than deserving of the title but still struggles with identity issues.

It is simple to associate a professional title with a doctor, a nurse, a lawyer, a banker, an accountant, an engineer, a teacher, an epidemiologist, a biochemist, a microbiologist, and the list goes on, but there is always the question of "with what title do I introduce myself in the field of public health without perhaps a prior widely recognized title?"

My colleague's suggestions were excellent. The first step is to believe in yourself and know that you have what it takes to be an expert. Don't let a conflict in the title make you doubt yourself.

Another approach to dealing with title identity crises is to associate your area of specialization with your name.

Community health, health policy and management, global health, biostatistics, health education, and epidemiology are just a few of the many specialties in public health. If you minored in health policy and management, you can confidently refer to yourself as a "public health administrator." You can call yourself a community health specialist or a health educator if you minored in community health or health education. Similarly, if you specialize in biostatistics, you can refer to yourself as a biostatistician or a public health biostatistician.

I know some of my readers may ask themselves, what if I am into community health, health education, and health policy? The answer to that is right in front of you.

You can either choose any of the specialization titles or just proudly and unapologetically call yourself a ''public health expert or specialist''.

Due to the highly flexible nature of the public health field, it is very possible to find yourself working in more than one of the aforementioned specialties. Rather than focussing on what title suits you best, go ahead, and leave a positive impression.

There is a local saying where I come from and that goes as follows;

A good palm wine taper does not need a signboard

Literally translated, this means that clients or customers seek you out or employ your services because of the high caliber of your work, not because of your position. In the field, numerous people are having an impact.

The last identity crisis, which I'd like to address partially here and partially in the following chapter, has to do with job offers. There are very few jobs that appear to be exactly "looking for public health personnel or something."

There is frequently this concern, particularly among newcomers to the field, about how to determine which job is best suited for them. Some job descriptions state that a degree in public health is a plus or is required, while others do not. At first glance, this may appear to be an identity issue, but upon closer inspection, you may need to reconsider your position.

The majority of public health training is meant to prepare you for a variety of positions. Some of the most common positions are monitoring and evaluation officer (also known as M&E), data analyst, health educator, community health officer, and health care administrator, to name a few (indeed, 2020).

If you wait for that specific job title with the headline "public health officer" before applying, you may become frustrated. However, it is important to note that, while your degree may qualify you for such positions, it is also necessary to take additional accredited courses to supplement your knowledge. We live in an ever-changing world where change and advancement are evident.

There are many more identity conflicts that may exist or be experienced that I did not mention in this chapter, but whatever that identity conflict is, it can be overcome. The first and most important step is to feel at ease and confident in the field of public health. In addition, remember that no matter what field or area you are in, there will always be challenges.

If it's any comfort, the majority of the mentors you have and admire have had some degree of identity conflict at some point in their lives. The most important thing, though is not to let go of the struggle, rather it is to identify and recognize the cause or trigger behind the conflict and take action to address it. If you put your mind to it, you can excel in your field.

CHAPTER 3

MONEY OR CAREER?

"A job is how you make money. A career is how you make your mark. A calling is how you acknowledge a higher version, whatever it may be" **Deepak Chopra**

I do not claim to be a financial analyst or a career expert, but there is one universally accepted fact. Some people devote their entire lives to chasing and slaving for money. Don't get me wrong: money is wonderful. Money, in fact, makes life easier and provides solutions to many of the problems we may face. However, Merriam-Webster defines a career as follows (Merriam-Webster, 2022):

"Career is a field for or pursuit of consecutive, progressive achievement especially in public, professional, or business life".

I underlined three crucial terms in the above definition: pursue, consecutive, and progressive.

In order to properly understand their relevance in both the advancement of our careers and the pursuit of financial security, let's try to analyze each of these phrases separately.

Pursuit can be defined as the act of chasing or tracking. To remain relevant in the field of public health, one must constantly pursue new ideas, new strategies, and new methods. As previously stated, we live in an ever-changing world. Never be satisfied with just a degree in public health. To become a public health expert in every sense of the term, one must constantly strive to stay relevant by going above and beyond and acquiring the necessary skills and training.

Consecutive means successive or most preferably back-to-back. There is no such thing as self-sufficiency or the feeling of "I know enough" when it comes to a career in public health or any other field. Keep yourself up to date to fully harness and maximize your career in public health. Every day, new inventions, theories, and diseases of public health concern emerge.

Modified methods of health education and community health intervention are available.

Being conservative and resistant to new and innovative methods that can advance your career will prevent you from becoming the public health expert you seek.

Progressive is interlinked with pursuit and being consecutive. I like to put it this way;

''The end result of pursuit and consistency should be progress''.

Always take a breather and ask yourself, "Am I making progress?" Am I on the right track with my skills and other activities to advance my career as a public health expert? Are they advantageous to me?

Many people believe that the highly regarded SWOT (Strengths, Weaknesses, Opportunities, and Threats) analysis is only useful for businesses and organizations, but this is not the case. The self-SWOT analysis is especially important in your career journey to determine whether you are just doing work or doing productive work.

After we've looked at the keywords in the definition of a career, let's see if there's a link between a career in public health and money.

There is no doubt that the current surge in the field of public health is due to many people believing it is a thriving industry with plenty of money (smiles). When I tell people I'm a public health expert, their reaction is almost always the same.

The smile comes first, followed by a mischievous grin, and most people would like to stop there, but not for others (laughs).

Some people will say, "Wow, public health is a great field with so many job opportunities." You appear to be quite young; how much do you earn? Can I easily find work if I change careers to public health? I've heard the pay package is competitive."

On one occasion, an acquaintance of mine told me he was going to enroll in an MPH program and then quit his job (mind you, he is one of the most prestigious and admirable professions in my country) to focus on public health because he was wowed by the salary offer on a public health-related job advertisement.

Yes, everyone pursues a career, a job, or whatever with the primary goal of making money. My question to you, the reader, is as follows:

''Are you seeking or are you in the public health career with the sole aim of making money or creating impact alongside?''

During the majority of my mentorship sessions with young people seeking advice in the field of public health. MONEY is always the most obvious motivator!

Many of them want to work in public health not for career opportunities, but for the money. I am not condemning the money motive, but in order to make a positive impact in this field, you must focus on developing your career.

There are currently many successful self-employed public health experts I know. They did not become very successful and financially secure by pursuing quick cash. Even, most of the organizations whose generous pay packages you admire often require more than just a degree in the public health degree. Every employer seeks value that extends far beyond passing an exam and having a degree. The goal of pursuing a career in public health should be more than just making money.

Expectations meet Reality

The truth is that people recognize and value expertise more than they do a job, just for money. The biggest surprise for most young public health professionals is finishing school, receiving their degree, and not being able to secure a good-paying job as they had hoped. All of their hopes of receiving that fat paycheck seem to vanish in a vast unending sea. Most of them, still highly disappointed, reluctantly resort to volunteering to gain experience, while others simply choose to further their education to avoid being idle. In the field, these are some of the harsh expectations that meet reality.

Grit is required in every line of work. Not everyone receives a job with a mouth-watering salary right after graduation.

Yes, there are employees who are willing to give fresh grads with no experience a chance in their business (kudos to such employers), but there are some employers who insist on the job experience before giving you a chance. A fun fact is that if your sole motivation for entering public health is financial gain, you are not alone. There are probably hundreds of thousands of people with the same goal. The big question is, "How do you then set yourself apart and distinguish yourself from the crowd?"

While pursuing my MPH, we had this one professor who always took the time to remind us that, while our program was dubbed a "professional master of public health," what will make us professionals is not that we did a professional master's program, but that we trained ourselves with the resources available to us to become professionals in the field.

Nobody becomes a professional by simply reading their lecture notes, especially in public health.
We are surrounded by numerous opportunities to hone our expertise in public health, some paid and others voluntary; having a growth mindset is essential if you intend to weather the storms.

Are you aware that people who have earned a Ph.D. or Doctorate in Public Health are still not considered qualified for certain jobs? Many people believe that if they continue their education and obtain a Ph.D., they will be able to obtain the job of their dreams. The answer to such a hypothesis, as I'd like to refer to it, can be YES or NO.

Yes, if you have a clear definition of who you want to become and have done the right research, you are confident getting that extra degree will be a great booster to your career.

No, if you do not have a clear rationale for pursuing that higher degree.

You can still pursue that Ph.D. degree and a holder of a master's degree in public health degree ends up being more qualified than you.

Interviews don't lie. There is a glaring difference between a qualified and well-informed applicant and a degree-certified applicant.

You can get all the degrees, certificates, and diplomas you want, but without a clear reason why you need them, they won't materialize and be useful to you.

In a conversation with an elderly friend, he inquired as to why I chose to pursue a Ph.D. in public health and what I planned to do with the certificate afterward. We started chatting, and as I was answering his question before I could finish, he said, 'then a short MBA course will be very useful to you.' I smiled unconsciously because he seemed to take the words right out of my mouth. Yes, in the long run, I will require MBA accreditation.

It is not urgent, but it is on my list of things I need to do to get where I want to go.

He also mentioned a few courses that might be of interest to me, and when I told him that I had already taken a few of them, he simply nodded in agreement.

The point of my sharing this brief interaction with my friend is not to tell you to go read every course on the planet (laughs) or to focus solely on formal education. I am also an entrepreneur, or "healthpreneur," which has helped my career tremendously. In conclusion, the message I am conveying is this: know where you are going.

When you don't have a clear direction, every course appears to be the best option.

With no clear direction, you may waste time doing things that add no value to the person you want to become. Of course, while having a clear direction, be flexible. Your expectations might occasionally conflict with reality, but that does not in any way mean you keep changing because things are changing. Rather, adjust your goals, modify the ones that require modification, and change the route if possible but don't lose sight of your intended destination.

CHAPTER 4

ENTREPRENEURSHIP

"The only way to do great work is to love what you do. If you haven't found it, keep looking. Don't settle. As with all matters of the heart, you will know when you find it"
Steve Jobs

Entrepreneurship is unquestionably one of the most popular topics in the twenty-first century. Gone are the days when people relied solely on monthly income from a 24/7 salary job that most of them did primarily out of financial necessity and with no other options. Entrepreneurship is the mother of all inventions today. People are starting to take calculated risks to pursue their true passions.

Entrepreneurship in public health can take many forms, including a profitable business venture, non-governmental organization (NGO), consultancy, writing, manuscript reviewing, data analysis, social media health influencers, and so on. Actually, one can make a living in more than one of these areas.

It is not unusual to come across an NGO founder who also works as a consultant and writer, or a public health specialist who uses social media to share helpful information.

In essence, there are numerous public health-related entrepreneurial fields in which you can work either full-time or part-time depending on your motivation and availability.

Many people start businesses without conducting proper research and gathering the necessary information to sustain them on their entrepreneurial journey. Being your own boss may seem appealing until the harsh reality of entrepreneurship hits you in the face.

Yes, when I started a health-based NGO with two of my friends at the time, we were incredibly passionate about providing health services to the community, giving back to the masses, and doing what we loved.

I remember the joy in our hearts when we were told over the phone that our registration documents had been signed and that we were now officially a registered non-profit health-related association under Cameroon's Ministry of Public Health.

Our first community project, which was entirely self-funded, was a huge success, and I felt more accomplished than ever (laughs). When I looked back and saw how excited I was, I knew I had made the right choice. Previously, I thoroughly enjoyed community health education, but the excitement and immediate successes diverted my attention away from more important matters.

Yes, we did open an NGO, but did we conduct adequate research on how to properly manage an NGO at the time? Were we going to always self-fund our projects?

Did we clearly define leadership roles to avoid future conflicts of interest, or did we believe that friendship would suffice? Did any of us receive formal grant and project writing training?

These are just a few of the questions I wish we had clear answers to at the start. Regardless, our desire to serve humanity in the field of health kept us going even during difficult times. I eventually took Agile/Scrum project management courses as well as grant writing classes. We are still fully operational and plan to expand in the coming years. Today I also double as a public health consultant and writer. I continue to acquire and improve my skills and methods to stay relevant. It has never been a smooth ride.

There are days I wake up feeling like I have made zero progress and other days I wake up feeling grateful. Both days are perfectly normal in the life of an entrepreneur. How you choose to react on both days will determine how far you will go.

You are the only one who knows what your purpose is. Things you do may not make sense to most people around you, but with your conviction and determination, when they see the results, they will begin to make sense.

I'm telling my side of the story because having a passion for something is NOT ENOUGH to sustain you as an entrepreneur. Having a purpose without clearly obtaining the necessary skills and training to achieve that purpose may work against you in the future.

Before venturing into any entrepreneurial field, ask questions from those who have already made a name for themselves in that domain, read books, google frequently asked questions about that field, seek the necessary knowledge, and most importantly, get the right mindset.

You may make it without stress, but the odds are that the success you seek may take years. Entrepreneurship is a worthwhile risk. It will require an investment of your time, money, and resources, as well as consistency and a lot of optimism, just like any other job. You cannot be afraid of what you do.

If you cannot conveniently package your services to people, no one will pick interest in you. If you do not try, you will spend your whole time guessing the what-ifs.

What is the worst that could happen? will you fail? What if you actually succeeded? How will you know if you do not try?

This is not to say that your first, second, or even third entrepreneurial venture will be a success. Some people have achieved success after several failed attempts. One thing that kept them going was the passion and commitment they had toward the goal they were pursuing.

Others pursue public health entrepreneurship on a part-time basis while working full-time jobs. They intend to use a portion of the revenue generated by these salary jobs to fund their entrepreneurial ventures, particularly those requiring a large amount of capital. These are some of the sacrifices made by people. Sometimes you only see the end result (success and fame) without realizing how much work and sacrifice went into it.

If I can leave you with one piece of advice, it is that you cannot afford to sit idle and do nothing with your degree. You didn't get all of that education to sit at home and mope. Get up and think!

There are so many things to do; all you have to do is look beyond your current situation. The success you seek is entirely dependent on you.

Consider a solution to the billions of health-related issues out there.

Ignore the opinions of the crowd, and ignore those who tried and failed once.

When it comes to public health, there is always something you can do. Get busy while you're looking for that dream job or on your way to becoming the person you want to be.

There are numerous national and international platforms in which I have been privileged to participate thus far in my public health journey, all thanks to the small efforts I have made. It makes no difference if you believe no one is paying attention to you or watching you; believe me, 'people are watching.

'All you may sometimes need to make significant growth or progress in your career is one opportunity, but how prepared are you when that opportunity finally appears?

 It is frequently stated;

''opportunity favors the one that is prepared''

Entrepreneurship is about taking calculated risks rather than random ones. Overcome your fear of failure and give it a shot; who knows what will happen?

"Your idea could be exactly what we all need without even realizing it."

CHAPTER 5

GO FOR IT

"Believe in yourself and Go for it. Whether it turns out good or bad, it was an experience. Be that person who decided to go for it" Adanze N. Cynthia

We've already talked a lot, and I am hoping that by now, you have an idea of what the public health field as an early or aspiring career looks like. In conclusion, whatever your expectations were, I only have two sentences for you;

If you are looking forward to starting a career in the field of public health, you have done the necessary research and are confident that is the path you want to take, GO FOR IT.

and

If you are already working in the field of public health, dear colleague, always bear in mind, that you are a professional, an expert in the field.

Always carry yourself as one.

Do not be rigid to changes.

Do not stop exploring opportunities to do better.

REFERENCES

Dhakal, R. (2020). Contribution of Social Science Disciplines to make Public Health Interdisciplinary. https://www.researchgate.net/publication/340077463_Contribution_of_Social_Science_Disciplines_to_make_Public_Health_Interdisciplinary

Elmer, J. (2019). Identity Crisis Definition, Symptoms, Causes, and Treatment. https://www.healthline.com/health/mental-health/identity-crisis#TOC_TITLE_HDR_1

indeed. (2020). Top 25 Public Health Careers (with Salaries and Job Descriptions) | Indeed.com. Indeed. https://www.indeed.com/career-advice/finding-a-job/public-health-careers

"Career." Merriam-Webster.com Dictionary, Merriam-Webster, https://www.merriam-webster.com/dictionary/career. Accessed 19 Sep. 2022.

Sako, S. N. (2011). Graduates Doing Menial Jobs Due To Unemployment – Cameroon Postline. Cameroon Post. https://cameroonpostline.com/graduates-doing-menial-jobs-due-to-unemployment/